35 EASY WAYS TO GET RID OF ACNE FAST

Marcia Savage

35 Easy Ways To Get Rid Of Acne fast

Copyright Information

Copyright © 2014 by Marcia Savage

Your Free Gift

As a way of saying thanks for your purchase, I'm offering a free guide that's exclusive to my readers.

In this guide, you will learn how to turn any messy room in into a nice, clean, and tidy room, cleaning in only 3 hours. Your home will stay clean every day and you will never have to worry about unexpected guests walking into a dirty house again. You can download this free report by going here.

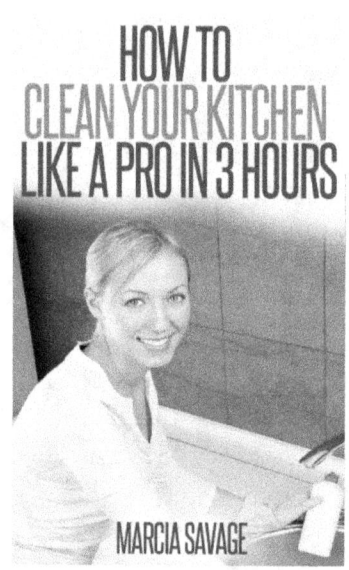

http://forms.aweber.com/form/76/315836976.htm

Table of Content

Regular Skincare Routine

If you follow regular skincare routine each morning, it will help maintain beautiful skin. Most skincare routines involve removing all oils and dirt from your pores with a deep cream cleaner, rinsing it with warm water, and applying moisture.

The first step in all skincare remedies is to wash your face. Washing your face in warm water will open pores for skincare treatments. There's no doubt about it, the best way to fight acne, blackheads, whiteheads, or pimples is to keep your skin clean. You should wash your face twice daily, in the morning and evening, to remove oils and dead skin build-up. After washing your face, apply astringent or toner for your skin type. People who have oily skin usually use astringent whereas people who have problems with dry skin uses toner.

Aside from washing your face, do not touch your face at all with your hands. Your hands produce oil and may have picked up dirt, which can be transferred to your face.

This also means that you shouldn't pop pimples with your hands, fingernails, or any other tool. Popping pimples this way will worsen the skin's issues, leading to acne scarring.

Acne is caused by different reasons. Hormonal changes are one reason, although this is more common with teenagers. However, too much cosmetics usage can be a reason for acne as cosmetics clogs the pores, which prevents your skin from breathing. Improper daily skincare and genetic factors are also causes for acne.

Hello! My name is Marcia Savage and just like most 30+ year old women, I have experienced acne, but I have an ace in the hole because my parents, aunts, uncles, grandparents, and their relatives had the same problems oily skin, the main culprit of acne. But they found natural home solutions that not only cured their acne, blackheads, whiteheads, and pimples, but also made their skin healthier, and sexy, fast. Do you want to cure acne? Do you want softer, sexier, and healthy skin in the next 30 days? Well, buckle your seat belt because we are about to go on one hell of a drive. Are you ready? Let's get started.

Cure Blackhead With Home Remedy 1

You'll need:

Toothpaste

3 Tbsp. of Salt

Plastic Spoon

Step One: Pour three tablespoons of salt into a bowl and add enough toothpaste to cover your face.

Step Two: Wash your face in hot water. Don't burn yourself! The water should be hot enough to open your pores because this helps the solution work.

Step Three: Using the back of the spoon, gently apply solution all over your face, and leave on for five minutes. Repeat the process at least twice a week for best results.

Cure Blackhead With Egg Mask 2

You'll need:

1 Egg

Face Brush

Tissue

Step One: Crack an egg, separate the yolk from white, and put the white in a bowl.

Step Two: Using your face brush, apply the egg white to your face, avoiding the eyes, nose, and mouth.

Step Three: Make a mask with the tissue. Cut out holes for your eyes, nose, and mouth and place it gently over your face

Step Four: Apply another layer of the egg white over the tissue and leave it on for 30 minutes.

Step Five: Gentle peel the tissue off your face in an upward direction.

Step Six: Wash your face in cold water.

If you have dry skin, repeat this process once a week; if you have oily skin, repeat twice a week.

You'll need:

1 Egg

1 Tbsp. Honey

2 Tbsp. Plain Flour

Face Brush

Step One: Crack the egg in a bowl, add one tablespoon of honey, and 2 tablespoon of plain white flour, and mix to a yogurt-like consistency.

Step Two: Using your face brush, apply the mixture to your face, avoiding your eyes, nose, and mouth. Leave the mixture on your face for 30 minutes.

Step Three: With a wash cloth, gently scrub the mask off your skin and rinse with cold water.

Eggs and honey will feed your skin, as the white flour exfoliates it, and honey works as an antibacterial agent.

You'll need:

1 Tbsp. Honey

2 Tbsp. Yogurt

Face Brush

Step One: Wash your face in warm water thoroughly.

Step Two: Pour yogurt and honey into a bowl, mix well, and apply mixture to your face with the face brush.

Step Three: Leave it on for 30 minutes to get the solution into your skin. After 30 minutes, rinse your face thoroughly with warm water. For best results, repeat this process twice a week.

You'll need:

1 Tbsp. Mineral Water

2 Tsp. Baking Soda

Face Brush

Step One: Pour mineral water in a bowl, add baking soda, and mix thoroughly to make a paste.

Step Two: Apply paste to your skin with the face brush and leave on for 25 minutes.

Step Three: After 25 minutes, rinse thoroughly with warm water.

Apply twice weekly as a bedtime moisturizer.

You'll need:

1 Tsp. Cinnamon Powder

1 Tsp. Lemon Juice

Step One: Pour cinnamon powder into a bowl and add one tablespoon of lemon juice. Mix into a paste.

Step Two: Apply solution onto your face with a face brush, and leave on 30 minutes.

Step Three: After 30 minutes, rinse with warm water. For best results, repeat this process two times a week.

You'll need:

1 Tsp. Honey

4 Whole Tomatoes

2 Tbsp. Oatmeal

Spoon

Blender

Step One: Cut up the tomatoes into small pieces and blend into a juice, add honey and oatmeal.

Step Two: Pour solution into a bowl and mix into a paste. Using your spoon, apply gently your face.

Step Three: Leave on for 20 minutes and rinse with warm water. Repeat this process 3 times weekly for best results.

You'll need:

½ Lemons

Cotton Balls

Step One: Squeeze ½ a lemon into a bowl, removing any seeds.

Step Two: Dip the cotton ball into the solution and wipe it on your face.

Step Three: Leave it on your face for 30 minutes and rinse off with warm water.

Lemon will not only remove acne but also brighten your skin.

Cure Whitehead With Baking Soda 2

You'll need:

3 Tbsp. Baking Soda

¼ cup of water

Face Brush

Step One: Pour the baking soda into the water and mix into a paste.

Step Two: Using your face brush, apply the mixture gently to your face. Be very careful around your eyes and nose.

Step Three: Leave on for 30 minutes and rinse off with warm water.

Baking soda will soak up all the oils and dirt out of your pores, leaving your skin nice and clean.

You'll need:

Potato flour

Cream

1 ripe Banana

Step One: In a bowl, mash your banana into a paste.

Step Two: Add two tablespoons of cream and mix well.

This is the milk cream I use. You can find it at Wal-Mart and it works best for dry skin. But any cream milk will do, just check your dairy department.

Step Three: Add one tablespoon of potato flour to the bowl and mix. Add enough flour and keep mixing until the solution becomes very dense. You can purchase potato flour at any of the follow sites.

http://www.nextag.com/Potato-Flour-Where-To-Buy/products-html?nxtg=19e10a3c051a-1BB8D026712442AB

Step Four: Apply the first layer to your skin and let dry. Then, apply a second layer.

Step Five: Leave the solution on for 30 minutes, and wash with warm water.

You'll need:

3 Aspirins

1 Tbsp. Water

Q-Tip

Step One: Crush the aspirin in a bowl, add one tablespoon of water, and mix to a paste.

Step Two: With a Q-Tip, apply the solution on to the scarred area, and leave it on for 20 minutes.

Step Three: After 20 minutes, rinse your face with warm water. Repeat this process 3 times weekly at bedtime for best results.

You'll need:

3 Aspirins

1 Tsp. Honey

1 Tsp. Lemon Juice

Step One: Crush the aspirin into a bowl and add honey and lemon juice. Mix into a paste.

Step Two: Apply paste to your skin with a spoon and leave it on for 20 minutes.

Step Three: After 20 minutes, rinse your face thoroughly with warm water. Repeat this process two times a week for best results.

You'll need:

1 Tbsp. Plain Yogurt

1 Tbsp. Turmeric

Face Pack Brush

Wet Tissue Wipe

You can find these items in most local grocery stores.

Step One: Clean your skin thoroughly with the wet tissue wipes.

Step Two: Mix one tablespoon of yogurt with one tablespoon of turmeric, and apply the mixture to your face.

Step Three: Wash the solution off your face with cold water after 30 minutes. Scrub the mask off your face with a wash cloth.

Apply this face mask twice weekly for the best results.

You'll need:

1 Egg

1 Tsp. Honey

Step One: Crack your egg, separate the white from the yolk, put the white in one bowl, and yellow in another. Add one teaspoon of honey in the white and mix well.

Step Two: Dip your finger into the solution and apply it to your face and leave it on for 15 minutes.

Step Three: After 15 minutes, wash off with warm water and blot dry with a clean towel. Apply the yellow to your face. This is a natural moisturizer and is good for your skin. After 15 minutes, rinse your face.

You'll need:

2 Tbsp. Honey

1 Tbsp. Olive Oil

4 Tbsp. Sugar

1 Tbsp. Lemon Juice

Step One: Mix the solution in a bowl and apply mixture to your face with a spoon.

Step Two: Massage solution gently into your skin for two minutes and rinse with warm water and blot your face dry with a clean towel.

For best results, repeat this process three times a week at bedtime.

You'll need:

Large Bowl

Hand Towel

Step One: Boil a large pan of water for 10 minutes. Take a dry towel and wipe off your face thoroughly.

Step Two: Pour the boiling water inside the bowl and let it sit for 2 minutes.

Step Three: Put the towel over your head and hang your head over the bowl. This will allow the stream from the hot water to open up the pores in your face, releasing any toxins in the skin.

You'll need:

1 Tbsp. Baking soda

1 Tsp. Peroxide

Step One: Pour baking soda and peroxide in a bowl, mix into a paste, and apply all over your face in a circular motion.

Step Two: Leave the mixture on for 10 minutes and rinse with warm water.

This solution helps to remove dead skin and dead skin blocks your pores, which leads to acne and other skin ailments.

You'll need:

1 Tbsp. Lemon Juice

1 Tbsp. Sugar

Step One: Pour solution into a bowl and mix thoroughly into a paste.

Step Two: Pour solution into your palm and apply it to your face. Leave it on for 20 minutes.

Step Three: After 20 minutes, rinse your face with warm water.

Repeat this process three times a week for best results.

You'll need:

3 strawberries

2 Tbsp. Vinegar

Step One: Cut up the strawberries into pieces, place in a bowl, and mash with a spoon. Add 2 tablespoon of vinegar and mix into a paste.

Step Two: Apply solution to your face and leave on for one hour.

Step Three: After one hour, rinse your face thoroughly with warm water.

You'll need:

2 Tbsp. Honey

2 Tbsp. Lemon Juice

Step One: Pour the honey in a microwave safe bowl and add lemon juice, place solution in the microwave on high for 5 minutes.

Step Two: After 5 minutes, remove the solution and let it sit for about 2 minutes and apply it to your face. Caution: don't burn yourself so test to be sure it is not too hot for your skin.

Step Three: Leave the solution on your face for 20 minutes and rinse with warm water.

You'll need:

Ice cubes

Hand Towel

Step One: Place ice cubes in a towel and wrap the towel around the cubes.

Step Two: Place the towel over the blemished area for 10 minutes.

You can use this daily because it will remove any swelling or redness cause by acne scars.

You'll need:

½ Cucumbers

½ Avocados

3 Tbsp. Lime Juice

3 Tbsp. Lemon Juice

½ cup water

Blender

Step One: Cut cucumber and avocado in half, remove the skins and seeds, cut into small pieces, and place in a bowl. Add lime and lemon to bowl, put in a blender, and add water. Blend to a paste.

Step Two: Apply solution to your face and leave on for 20 minutes and rinse with warm water.

This mask is great for your skin so repeat the process three times a week for best results.

You'll need:

3 Bags Green Tea

Paper Towel

Step One: Put tea bags in a bowl and add boiling water. Leave the bags in until the tea cools down. Remove the bags but don't throw them away.

Step Two: Place the paper towel into the tea. Let it become good and wet and apply it to your face. Don't get it in your eyes or mouth. Leave it on your face for 30 minutes and gently pull away.

Step Three: Rinse your face with warm water. You can use the tea bags for the next acne mask.

Cure Acne With Tea And Lemon Mask 10

You'll need:

3 Tea Bags

1 Tbsp. Lemon Juice

Step One: This solution is only for people with oily skin. Cut open the 3 bags on green tea and add them to the bowl of tea, add one tablespoon of lemon juice, and mix to a paste.

Step Two: Apply the mixture to your skin, massage into your face gently, in a circular motion, and leave it on for 20 minutes.

Step Three: After 20 minutes, rinse with warm water.

You'll need:

3 Green Tea Bags

1 Tbsp. Honey

This solution is for people with dry skin. It safe to use 3 times a week.

Step One: Cut open the three tea bags and pour them in the cup of tea. Add one tablespoon of honey and mix to a paste.

Step Two: Apply the solution onto your skin, carefully avoiding the eyes and nose. Leave the mixture on for 20 minutes and rinse with warm water.

You'll need:

2 Tbsp. Lemon Juice

2 Tbsp. Castor Oil

2 ½ Tbsp. Honey

½ cup Sugar

Step One: Pour the sugar in a bowl and add castor oil, honey, and lemon juice and mix well.

Step Two: Apply the mixture to your face and gently massage for two minutes. Leave the solution on for 20 minutes.

Step Three: After 20 minutes, rinse your skin with cool water. Repeat the process 4 times a week for two weeks for best results.

You'll need:

1 Medium Potato

Peering Knife

Towel

Step One: Slice the potato in thin slices with your peering knife and put them in a bowl.

Step Two: Lay the towel over your pillow put on some soft music, lay down face up and put the sliced potato all over your face. Leave the potato on for 45 minutes.

Step Three: After 45 minutes remove the slices and wash your face in cold water.

You'll need:

2 Tbsp. Cocoa Butter

Step One: Wash your hands and face with warm water and blot dry with your towel.

Step Two: Apply cocoa butter all over your face and leave on for 1 ½ hours.

Step Three: After 1 ½ hours rinse, with warm water.

Cocoa butter has a miraculous effect on acne and is the perfect solution for healing it. It is the perfect solution to use nightly, if you have dry skin.

Cure Acne Scars With Banana Mask 4

1 Banana

Bowl

Step One: Wash your face in warm water and blot dry with a towel.

Step Two: Cut banana in, half place in a bowl, and, with a spoon, smash into a paste.

Step Three: Apply banana mask on your face and leave on for one hour.

Step Four: After one hour, rinse away the mask with warm water. Repeat this process 4 times a week for best results.

You'll need:

2 Tbsp. White Vinegar

Bowl

Step One: Wash your face with cold water and apply a small amount of vinegar on the affected area.

Step Two: Leave the solution on for half an hour then clean off with cold water and blot dry.

White vinegar is great for people with oily skin. It will also light dark spots on your skin caused by acne scars. You should use it twice weekly for best results.

You'll need:

1 banana

Hand Towel

Step One: Peel a banana. Take the peel and cut into two inch slices.

Step Two: Wash your face in warm water and rub the inner side of the peel over the affected area. Leave it on for 20 minutes and rinse with warm water.

Banana is an amazing skincare solution. It also reduces winkles, whitens your teeth, and is safe to use daily.

You'll need:

Mint leaves

1 Tbsp. Lemon Juice

1 Tsp. Turmeric

Step One: Grind a handful of mint leaves, one tablespoon lemon juice, and one teaspoon turmeric powder. Mix into a paste.

Step Two: Rub paste onto your pimples and let dry.

Step Three: Wash thoroughly with warm water and blot dry. Repeat this process two times a week for best results.

Cure Pimple With Herbs 2

You'll need:

1 Tbsp. Sandalwood Powder

2 Tbsp. Rose Water

Step One: Add the solution into a bowl and mix into a paste.

Step Two: Rub paste onto the affected area and leave on overnight.

Step Three: Rinse solution off with warm water in the morning and blot dry.

You can find these products at your local health food store.

Cure Pimples With Vicks Vapor Rub

You'll need:

1 Tbsp. Vicky Vapor Rub

Wash Cloth

Step One: Wash your face with cold water and blot dry with a hand towel.

Step Two: Apply vapor rub to the affected area and leave on overnight.

Step Three: The next morning, rinse off the solution with warm water.

It very important not to get the vapor rubs in your eyes, nose, or mouth. After using the vapor rub, wash your hands thoroughly several times.

Cure Pimples With Cinnamon

You'll need:

3 Tbsp. Honey

3 Tsp. Cinnamon

Step One: Pour three teaspoon of cinnamon into a bowl, add three tablespoon of honey, and mix.

Step Two: Apply the mix to your skin as a moisturizer twice a day, once in the morning and in the evening.

Step Three: Leave on your skin for 30 minutes and rinse thoroughly with warm water and blot dry.

Cure Pimples With Orange Peels

You'll need:

2 Oranges

1 Carton of Plain Yogurt

Step One: Peel two oranges and let the peels dry. Grind the dried orange peel, mix in with small packet of yogurt, and apply to your face and leave for one hour.

Step Two: After one hour, rinse your face with warm water.

This mixture is a moisturizer and is safe to use daily if you have dry skin, or three times a week if you have oily skin.

www.ingramcontent.com/pod-product-compliance
Lightning Source LLC
Chambersburg PA
CBHW052016280526

45793CB00005B/1003

* 9 7 8 1 4 9 9 2 3 5 4 3 2 *